# Six Strategies *to be a* More Effective *and* Efficient Monitor

A practical personal approach to monitoring clinical trials

Patricia O. Kasper, MS, CCRA

PKASPER & ASSOCIATES
CLINICAL RESEARCH TRAINING AND OPERATIONS

Learn to Grow®

Published by Patricia O. Kasper

Six Strategies to be a More Effective and Efficient Monitor
Paperback Edition


Printed in the United States of America

ISBN Number: 978-0-9862191-1-5

# Table of Contents

# Introduction

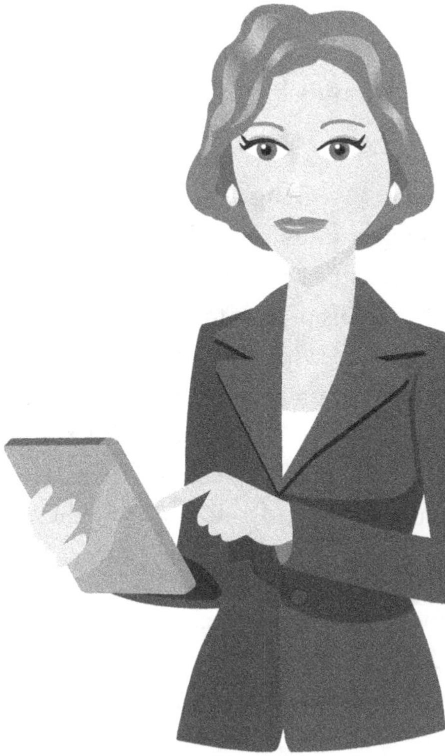

**Monitoring clinical trials is the core of what** clinical research associates (CRAs) or monitors do every day. Because few formal classes are available to train you to do this work, most of the skills are learned by doing. It is an apprentice-style career. Yet we all know that learning on the job can be painful at times. What can you do to speed up the learning process?

If you are lucky, an experienced monitor will work closely with you and show you the skills you need. But it is much harder today to find mentors to help new monitors. Workshops and classroom courses provide training on the fundamentals of clinical research, FDA regulations, and some specific tasks such as how to write a monitoring report. Yet, few resources are available that truly teach you how to conduct a monitoring visit.

From years of experience working as a director in clinical research and mentoring many monitors, I found that most CRAs—despite having attended industry workshops—still have gaps in their knowledge of the specific details of how to effectively and efficiently conduct a monitoring visit. To address this need, I developed formal training classes. With a passion for mentoring and education, I trained many individuals over the past two decades and observed a common thread among these students—most seemed to lack essential skills in the same areas. As a result, I found myself repeating the same points over and over again.

I decided to document some of the techniques I was teaching both at monitoring sites and in training workshops. From these notes and ideas, I developed this book that is short and to the point. It is designed to help CRAs acquire some of the specific skills needed to improve performance and increase efficiency when monitoring at clinical research sites.

## My Story about a Monitoring Disaster

While working as a senior CRA, I was asked to accompany a less experienced CRA on a site visit because her manager was worried about her poor performance and lack of follow-up. We planned the day trip and flew off to the site. Sitting next to each other on the plane, we discussed her plans for the visit. I asked her some questions about the protocol, the agenda, and strategies for interacting with the coordinator. Not good. She was not prepared.

I did what I could to get us ready for the day, and when we arrived at the site, we tackled the business of reviewing charts and checking case report forms (CRFs). There were numerous dosing errors, two protocol violations, and many data queries that were still outstanding from the last site visit. The regulatory binder was a mess, and she did not interact well with the study coordinator or the principal investigator (PI). In short, it was a rough day.

This junior CRA made many mistakes and demonstrated a huge lack of understanding about what to do and how to do it. I had not seen this behavior from her in the office, so I was surprised by how poor her performance was in the field. During our debrief session, I discovered many of the reasons for this lack of competency and worked closely with her to improve her monitoring skills.

# Summary of the Six Strategies to be a More Effective and Efficient Monitor

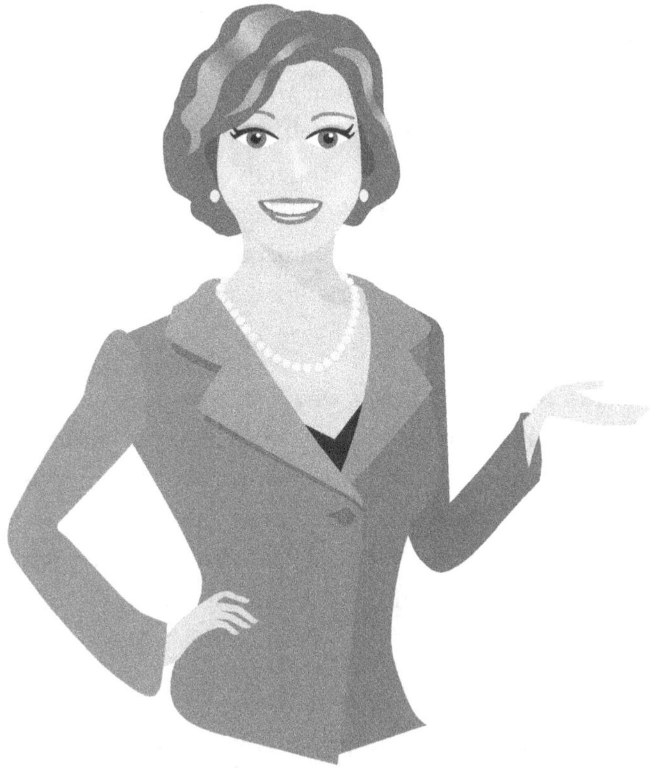

In this book, I will share many of the techniques I gave to this inexperienced CRA. Write down the ones that work best for you.

### Bulleted checklist

At the back of this chapter is a short, bulleted summary of all the techniques described here. You may want to use it as your own personal checklist to become an exceptional monitor.

### References

A list of some of the most relevant references to regulations and guidelines used in monitoring clinical trials are provided at the end of the book. Look these up on-line and become familiar with the topics relevant to you to become a more informed monitor. While there are numerous ways to enter the field of clinical research, many individuals come into monitoring with a degree in life sciences or medical sciences. Training in scientific data collection and management methods is valuable to ensure site compliance with the research study protocol and all regulations. Yet, to be truly effective in the role, CRAs must also have good project and people management skills. These methods and techniques for planning and managing time, objects, and people will help you accomplish the myriad of tasks required to monitor a clinical trial.

I will start by giving reasons why it is so important to monitor properly. By focusing on the "why," many CRAs are better able to understand the nuances of the business. Unfortunately, most of the regulations are vague, and many times CRAs need to use good judgment to determine the best way to document a situation. By thinking through the reasons why monitoring is important and seeing some of the consequences of poor monitoring, you will improve your monitoring skills.

Next, I will give you techniques to increase your efficiency and effectiveness during any phase of an investigational drug trial or any class of a medical device study.

Much of what has become industry standard and accepted practice is acquired through experience. Based on my years of experience as a CRA, manager, and director, I will provide techniques to help you monitor clinical investigations more effectively and efficiently. Along with these techniques, I will share the methods—the keys to success—to implement these techniques. To make these ideas come alive, I have included personal stories to highlight each technique.

The following are the six techniques discussed in this book:

- **Anticipate:** Consider all the things that could go wrong before and during your monitoring visit. Make a checklist to keep track of all these details.
- **Prepare:** Learn all you can about the protocol, the product, and the regulations.
- **Prioritize:** Know the most important tasks that must be accomplished. Determine how much time you expect each task to take and allocate a reasonable amount of time to complete each one. Create a priority plan and a backup plan to accomplish these tasks and adhere to that plan.
- **Organize:** Create an organizational system that works for you and stick with it.
- **Scrutinize:** Keep track of the myriad of numbers, dates, facts, and names. Have checklists for each area reviewed.
- **Follow up:** Have a rock-solid system for tying up loose ends after every visit.

Finally, I will provide an example of a warning letter from the Food and Drug Administration (FDA) citing Pfizer's failure to follow the regulations and the resulting consequences of improper monitoring. From this warning letter, we can learn how to implement systems and procedures that help ensure proper monitoring for clinical trials from the beginning.

I enjoy training, mentoring, and helping CRAs learn how to function more effectively and efficiently. I have taught in many different ways: one-on-one, small seminars, and larger conference sessions. This interest in training led me to write a book in order to help monitors understand the reasons why monitoring is so important and learn specific techniques to become a better monitor.

It was purely by coincidence that I entered the field of clinical research. After working as a medical technologist, I received my master's degree and worked in a basic research laboratory. While doing this bench work I just happened to read about an internal CRA position. It sounded fabulous. I could envision doing the job because it was a terrific blend of my medical technology knowledge and my experience in the laboratory. Also, I would get to travel and conduct research on new drugs. Wow! What an opportunity. After persevering, I finally got a job as a CRA where I received one day of training from the woman who was leaving the position.

I know how it feels to be thrown into the deep end without a clear understanding of what a monitoring visit requires and how to tackle those requirements.

By reading this book you will learn how to make monitoring easier, more efficient, and more enjoyable for you.

## Summary Checklist of the Six Strategies to be a More Effective and Efficient Monitor

| | Strategy | Key |
|---|---|---|
| ✔ | **ANTICIPATE** Consider all the things that could go wrong before and during your monitoring visit. | **KEY** Create a ***Reminder Checklist*** for each site visit to keep track of all these details. |
| ✔ | **PREPARE** Learn all you can about the protocol, the product, and the regulations. | **KEY** Make ***Spreadsheets*** for all the important areas of review. |
| ✔ | **PRIORITIZE** Know the most important tasks that must be accomplished and have a plan to accomplish them. | **KEY** Generate a ***Priority Plan*** and a ***Back-up Plan.*** |
| ✔ | **ORGANIZE** Create an organizational system that works for you and stick with it. | **KEY** Build a ***Color-coded*** system for all documents associated with each area. |
| ✔ | **SCRUTINIZE** Keep track of the myriad of numbers, dates, facts, and names. Have checklists for each area reviewed. | **KEY** Construct a ***Zip List*** spreadsheet for tracking data at the site visit. |
| ✔ | **FOLLOW UP** Have a rock-solid system for tying up loose ends after every visit. | **KEY** Produce an ***Action Item Table*** after every site monitoring visit and ensure it is completed. |

# Importance of Good Monitoring

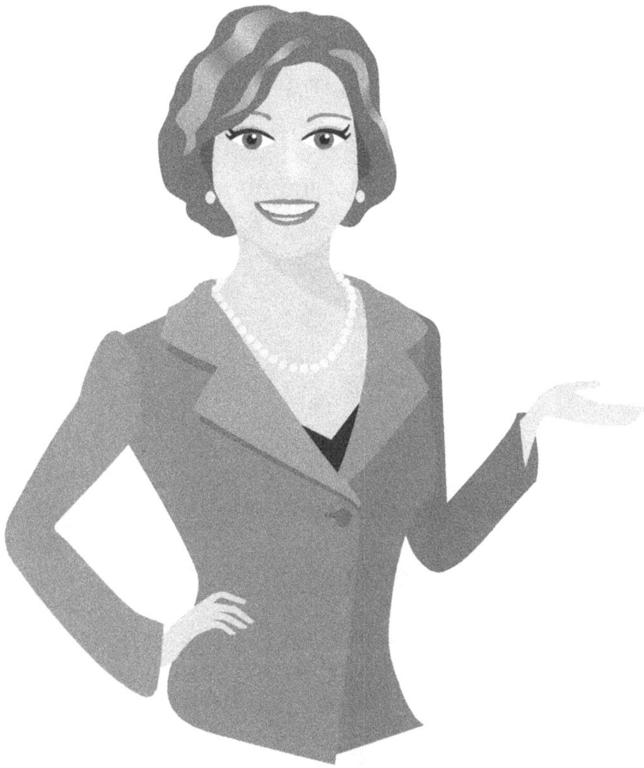

**As clinical monitors, we are tasked to review** the safety of patients and ensure accurate, high-quality data. In order to do that, we need to understand the regulations and have techniques that allow us to function quickly, decisively, and correctly at each site monitoring visit.

NOTE: For reference, the key regulations and guidelines for monitors are listed at the end of the book.

New clinical monitors are always astonished to find that the regulations provide little information on how to perform their duties. The FDA regulations indicate what tasks are required but not how to perform them. For example, 21 CFR 312.56(a) states: "The sponsor shall monitor the progress of all clinical investigations being conducted under its IND." Unfortunately, it doesn't statehow to monitor the progress of clinical investigations. Much of what has become industry standard and accepted practice needs to be acquired through experience.

There is so much more involved in monitoring such as:

1. How often do we monitor?
2. What data should we review?
3. How do we fix mistakes?
4. How do we handle non-compliance?
5. Which regulatory documents must be maintained?
6. How do we track what we have done?
7. What is good documentation practice?
8. What are all the parameters of product accountability?

These are some of the nuances of proper monitoring. In addition to learning the laws and guidelines, an understanding of the reasons why efficient monitoring is so beneficial helps clarify the detailed tasks. Here are some of the reasons why monitoring accurately is so important:

**It's the law.** This is a regulated environment, so we are under an obligation to follow the laws. The only way to do this is to learn the applicable laws and guidelines and learn the industry standards that apply to these laws. If a law is broken, a citation may occur. The results can be a Form 483 Inspectional Observations issued by FDA, a warning letter, a court case, a disqualification, jail time, and/or a monetary fine.

**We care about patients.** Many sick patients are enrolled in clinical trials and are treated with investigational products or medical devices. We need to ensure that safety information is collected quickly and correctly so that the safety profiles of these investigational drugs or devices can be known as soon as possible.

**We are scientists.** We want to know about the product we are testing; therefore, we need good clean data in real time. Of course, the blind is not broken in a randomized blinded trial until the end of the study, but data are collected on an ongoing basis for reports and data listings. When we clean the data as it is collected, there are fewer outstanding queries to be resolved at the end of the trial.

**We need to save time and money.** The drug and medical device development industry is becoming astronomically expensive. Anything that is done to save time and money will benefit the company, the patients, and society as a whole. It is our obligation to do so. Doing it right the first time is the best way to ensure high quality at the lowest cost.

Think about these reasons as you read this book, and it will motivate you to become even more proficient at your job.

# Anticipate

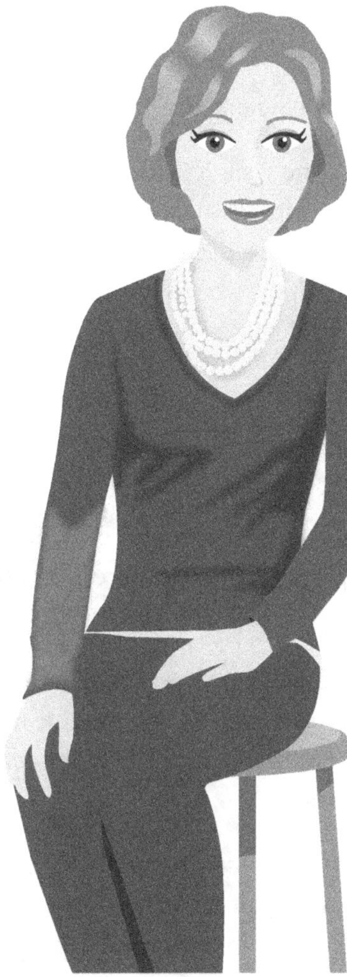

Before you go on a monitoring trip, you need to anticipate all the needs and challenges and be prepared for them. A good way to approach this is to think about the potential issues that could occur during your site visit.

Ask yourself, "What could go wrong?" This isn't a negative attitude but rather an experienced monitor's perspective. If you anticipate potential problems, it is easier to deal with them. Some issues are relatively easy to anticipate and avoid. Other issues are much harder to predict, but if you have a plan or an idea about how you might handle a problem, you will be more efficient and effective when it occurs.

When planning your site visit, it is important to consider potential issues before scheduling a trip. Identify areas that can be handled offsite through teleconferences such as discussing ongoing issues or adverse event rates. These topics can then be followed up at the site without consuming too much time during the visit.

*Here are a few issues related to the site, the people, and the data:*

## Site Issues

During an on-site visit, you may encounter challenges related to weather, parking, timing, space, internet access, or other factors. Here are some examples:

- If there are storms predicated for the area, flying in that morning and making it to your appointment on schedule may be problematic. In that case, book a flight that arrives the night before so you can be ready to start promptly at 8:00 a.m.
- If you are visiting a large medical center, it will likely have a huge parking lot. To ensure that you arrive on schedule, allow extra time in case you need to circle the lot to find a parking space or walk to the office from blocks away.
- If you are visiting a geographical area that does not have reliable internet connectivity, you may not be able to count on transmitting data or documents back to the sponsor. In this case, you may need to make copies and hand-carry or ship them.

By anticipating these kinds of issues, you can arrange ways to manage the potential problems.

## My Story about Anticipating

Several years ago, I asked the CRA whom I was training to arrange the logistics for an on-site visit, including the flights and appointment times. We were going from San Francisco to Los Angeles for a one-day monitoring visit. When she told me she had scheduled an 8:00 a.m. flight, I knew we needed to talk.

I reviewed the timeline with her. If we took the 8:00 a.m. flight, by the time we picked up our rental car and drove to the site in the morning rush-hour traffic, we would not arrive before 11:00 a.m. The CRA then realized that we had to take the 6:30 a.m. flight which required getting up at 4:00 a.m. to drive to the airport, park, get through security, and be at the gate by 6:00 a.m. Wow, what a difference!

When we arrived at the site at 9:00 a.m., the Principal Investigator (PI) informed us that he was closing the office at 2:00 p.m. that day due to an unexpected situation. By working as fast as we could and skipping lunch, we were able to do an acceptable day's work. Imagine what the manager would have said if we had arrived at 11:00 a.m. and left at 2:00 p.m.?

## People Issues

People issues—such as an overworked clinical research coordinator (CRC), new staff members, or a coordinator with personal problems—can impact the amount of time you will need with each person and the actual work you can accomplish during the visit.

By considering the people at the site, you can anticipate when you may need to train a new hire, coach a junior coordinator, or help someone who is overworked. When I am monitoring, I always allow some time in the day to deal with people issues. Make a few minutes to answer questions, hear about problems or get to know your colleagues a little better. By knowing the people and their troubles and triumphs, you can become a more effective monitor.

The business philosophy "It's all about the people" certainly applies to the work of a monitor. No matter what else you do—it's always about the people because the people are doing the work. They read the protocol, find the patients, enter the data, become angry when things don't go well, and work harmoniously when they feel appreciated. In order to get a high-performing team and good quality data, you need to connect with the people at the site and at the sponsor.

Monitors now are expected to accomplish more in less time so they often do not have time to spend in casual conversation. My suggestion is to use a few minutes at the beginning of each day to discuss the clinical protocol and status of the study with the appropriate individuals. This will ensure that you get to know the people doing the work. If you don't have much time for chats then make sure each discussion is focused on the project, recruitment, investigational product, issues, problems, solutions, or questions directly related to understanding and completing the protocol.

When you have found the time to have a discussion make sure you give that person your undivided attention. Since you only have a few minutes, make sure you make eye contact with them the entire time you are talking together. Do not glance at your phone, computer, or watch. This is not only rude but it distracts you from the conversation. Focus on what the individual is saying, repeat back what you have heard, and make some notes if necessary to capture all the important elements of the discussion.

Find ways to connect with each person involved with the trial at the site. An effective technique is to keep short notes: what they like and don't like, who is new, or who has special pet peeves. I jot down this information in my smart phone or tablet and review these details prior to each site visit. I can't remember every fact about the site personnel, but by doing some homework in advance I can refresh my memory on details about each individual. Anticipating issues and connecting with each person facilitates a smoother site visit.

Find out information about the site staff and keep track of these details to help you connect with the people.

## Data Issues

Good clean data are imperative for good quality trials. Review the monitoring plan, spreadsheets and data listings in advance to help you anticipate issues with the data before you arrive at the site. Here are some typical issues you may encounter with data at trial sites:

- Too much data to review is a common complaint from monitors. If this is the case at the site, determine which data will get the most attention. Focus on safety first, then review other data points that are critical to the study or were requested by the study team. Use the monitoring plan as the guide for exactly what should be reviewed during each site visit.

- Sites with many queries are problematic because it usually means that the entire staff is either confused, overworked, poorly trained, or disorganized. A site with lots of queries needs extra attention during your monitoring visit. Find out the root cause of the numerous queries before you go on-site by reviewing data remotely, if possible.

If the coordinator is confused, spend time clarifying the issues; if overworked, determine if it is possible to provide him or her with more support; if poorly trained or disorganized, add in training time. Determine ways to ensure that fewer queries are generated in the future.

- A complicated protocol with a myriad of procedures and a long list of requirements will take more time to monitor. Anticipate these site visits will take longer. Schedule accordingly.
- A site with several protocol violations is a red flag, so schedule time to discuss these violations with the coordinator and the PI during the site visit. Protocol violations can signal poor compliance with good clinical practice (GCP), a lack of understanding of the protocol, or inadequate training of the staff.

These kinds of data issues are all common in this business. By paying attention to the data, reviewing data listings, and knowing what data are the most important, you can anticipate where the complications will be and where you should spend most of your time.

## Key to Success to Anticipate

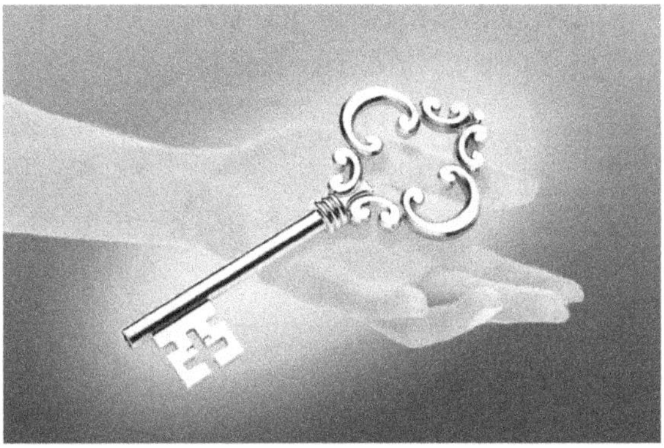

### Create a Reminder Checklist for each site visit.

Use this checklist to track notes and information about what to anticipate at each site. Write down issues about the site, the people, the data, or any areas that concern you. These are your own personal notes and are not included in the Trial Master File or a trip report. Even though these are your own notes, be very objective and only include facts (never opinions or negative comments) on this checklist.

I recommend creating a Reminder Checklist in a table format with a small box on the left and a section for notes on the right. Color code each section to stay organized. Go through the list and check off the areas for the upcoming visit. This will remind you of various facts and focus your efforts where they are needed the most.

## Example: Reminder Checklist*

### Dr. J.P. San Diego, CA, Study XYZ Site 621

| | Site Issues |
|---|---|
| | Parking problems, use lot 5B or arrive before 8 a.m. if parking in lot 1A |
| | **People Issues** |
| | Marge C. out on maternity leave July 1, identify replacement coordinator & plan to train |
| | Dr. J.P. not available on Tuesdays |
| | Research pharmacy appts better before 2 p.m. Pharmacist Stephanie M. recently graduated from UCLA |
| | **Data Issues** |
| | Request safety report data listing from Kim L. at least 5 business days prior to site visit |

*All names in this example are fictional.

# Prepare

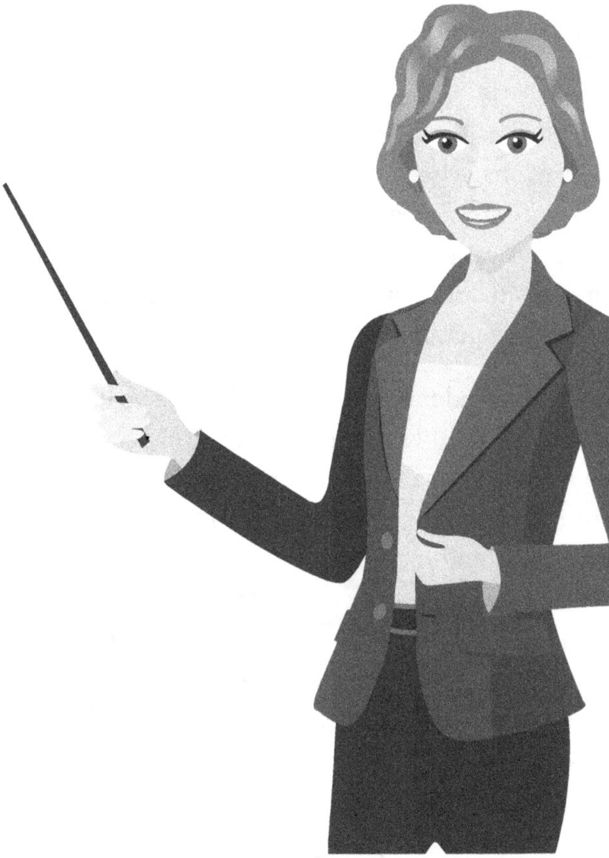

In order to be credible and professional, you need to prepare thoroughly before each site visit. Think about the last time you attended a meeting where the speaker came prepared with an agenda, documents, references, and facts. Were you impressed by the speaker's professionalism? Did the preparation bolster the speaker's credibility and perceived competence?

As you prepare for a site visit, use this same technique and allow as much time as necessary to get ready for the trip. Include enough time in your schedule to anticipate potential issues for each site and prepare to handle each one expeditiously. This preparation time will contribute significantly to your credibility, professionalism, and overall success.

Before a site visit, consider what kinds of questions need to be answered or what areas have been problematic in the past and structure your preparation accordingly. Preparation comes in many forms. Of course, the kind of preparation needed for a site visit will depend on various issues and the situation, but there are several important areas in which CRAs can improve performance if these tools are implemented.

Prepare a site visit agenda. Before going on a site visit, send an agenda to the site coordinator to identify the meeting objectives and get agreement on the specific tasks that will be completed during the visit. When preparing the agenda, be sure to consider what was covered in the prior visit and include details of what is planned for the upcoming meeting. By providing a clear list or table of the patient charts that will be reviewed, the regulatory documents that must be available, and whom you expect to see during the day, you will have a more efficient visit. It is helpful to include an estimate of the time needed for each task, your expected arrival and departure times, and planned lunch break. This well thought-out preparation will help you as well as the site personnel.

## My Story about Preparing

When I first started as a CRA, there was a site in Maryland that taught me a big lesson about being prepared. I flew in the day before the site visit from the West Coast, drove to a nearby hotel, and crashed that night. In the morning I had jet lag and was moving slowly. I grabbed a quick breakfast, found my rental car in the parking lot in the pouring rain, and navigated through rush hour traffic to the site. I arrived about five minutes before my scheduled appointment, and, of course, did not review the protocol or my notes. After all, I had conducted several monitoring visits for this protocol and thought I knew it well.

After exchanging a few pleasant words with the Principal Investigator (PI), he began asking me questions about the logistics of the protocol. His staff was having problems scheduling the required tests in the sequence required in the protocol. When he asked me a question, I would refer to my notes and either answer his question or say, "Oh, I will have to get back to you on that." This continued for over fifteen minutes, and I could tell he was not getting the answers he needed.

Finally, the PI indicated that he had patients to see, got up to leave the room, turned around at the door and stated, "When you have the answers to help us implement this protocol, kindly provide them to me." The experience taught me a valuable lesson: most physicians are very quick minded, want answers immediately, and will not wait around for a junior CRA to get her act together. I learned to prepare, prepare, prepare so that I would not end up in that situation again!

## Example Agenda*

### Dr. J.P. San Diego, CA, Study XYZ Site 621

| Contact Person | Topic | Time | Location |
|---|---|---|---|
| Steven H., CRC | Sign in, get daily password, discuss plans for the day | 8:30 – 9:00 am | Steven's desk #1144 |
| N/A | Review charts for pts # 3218-3229 | 9:00 – 12:00 noon | Monitoring room #1145 |
| Lunch | N/A | 12:00 – 12:30 p.m. | Magnolia Café |
| Dr. J.P. Principal Investigator | Review status of protocol. Discuss payment schedule. | 12:30 – 1:00 p.m. | Dr. P's office #1148 |
| N/A | Review eCRFs for pts # 3218-3229 and outstanding data queries | 1:00 – 2:30 p.m. | Monitoring room #1145 |
| Stephanie M., Pharmacist | Review product accountability records | 2:30 – 3:30 p.m. | Research Pharmacy, Bldg 7, room 019 |
| N/A | Review regulatory binder | 3:30 – 4:00 p.m. | Monitoring room #1145 |
| Steven H., CRC | Discuss issues and questions. Schedule next visit. | 4:00 – 5:00 p.m. | Steven's desk #1144 |

*All names in this example are fictional.

**Review the prior monitoring report.** If you are monitoring several sites or several different protocols, there are many tasks to juggle. Focus your attention on one site at a time and closely examine that site's issues. Before visiting the site, review the monitoring reports and action items from prior visits. Look at what items were covered during the visits. Review the charts that were monitored. Examine the areas that were left undone and figure out if they still need attention. Determine if there are any outstanding items so you can address them during the visit. All of this analysis will enable you to spend your time on the most important areas.

**Review the data for that site.** To effectively review data, you need to request data listings or run reports using the electronic data capture (EDC) system. The types of data vary by protocol, but critical reports— ones that include screen failures, patient enrollment, adverse events, missed visits, protocol violations, or patient dropouts—can help you isolate problem areas and identify where you should focus your attention during your next monitoring visit. Remember, you are responsible for ensuring that the data are accurately transcribed into the CRFs. You are also responsible for checking that all the patients are valid and that the site continues to follow the protocol. Data listings are effective tools to help you review the data efficiently and meet your responsibilities.

**Pay attention to the exact requirements of the protocol.** While reading electronic documents, it helps to bookmark important sections such as synopsis, objectives, schedule of events, and adverse events so they can be retrieved quickly. To capture the most important points, highlight key areas of the protocol. I encourage CRAs to actually memorize crucial areas of the protocol such as the inclusion/exclusion criteria, key efficacy endpoint measurements, and the most common adverse events. This kind of knowledge goes a long way establishing your credibility and dedication to that clinical protocol. It separates experienced monitors from junior ones.

**Understand the investigational product.** Understanding the investigational product is another area that needs your attention. It is your responsibility to know the dosing requirements of the drug or the instructions for use for a device, the temperature for storing the product, the timing for dispensing it, and every detail about completing the investigational product accountability forms. You should understand the mechanism of action and most important side effects that may occur based on the animal data reported in the investigator's brochure. All of these little facts about the protocol should be on hand prior to a monitoring visit. Spreadsheets are a necessity so that all the details are readily available.

## Key to Success to Prepare

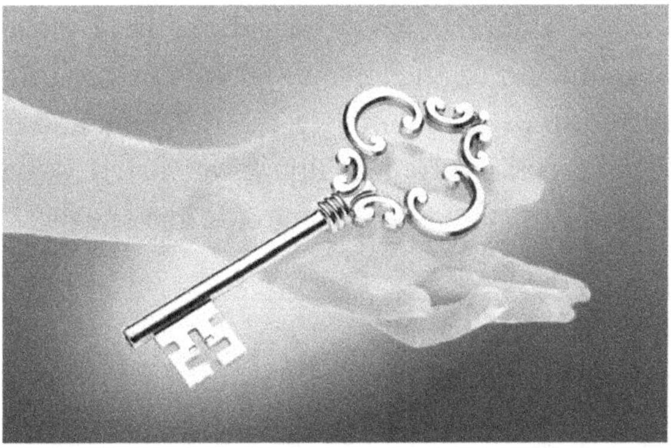

### Create Spreadsheets for all the important areas of review.

Make appropriate spreadsheets for all the areas you plan to examine during the site visit. Utilizing the spreadsheets will ensure that you are well prepared for your site visit.

Here are examples of various types of spreadsheets that are useful during your monitoring visit. If you are using an electronic data capture (EDC) system then use these listings from that system. If there is not an EDC system you may need to create your own:

- Dosing requirements
- Visit schedules
- Required lab specimens
- Timing of pharmacokinetic (PK) samples to be drawn
- Prohibited medications or procedures
- Serious adverse events or unanticipated adverse device effects

Below is an example of a dosing spreadsheet. In this example patients are dosed at 3.5 mg/kg. Create the spreadsheet by labeling it for the study and site number, enter the patient numbers, and enter the weight in kilograms. Set up the formula in the third column of cells to automatically multiply the patient's weight by 3.5 mg and the amount of drug to be dispensed will automatically be calculated. Leave a column for notes to capture any issues with dosing at that site.

## Dosing Requirements

**Dr. J.P. San Diego, CA,**

**Study XYZ Site 621**

| Pt Number | Pt weight kg | Dose in mg | Dosing Notes 3.5 mg/kg |
|---|---|---|---|
| 621-01 | 52 | 182 | |
| 621-02 | 89 | 311.5 | |
| 621-03 | 97 | 339.5 | |

# Prioritize

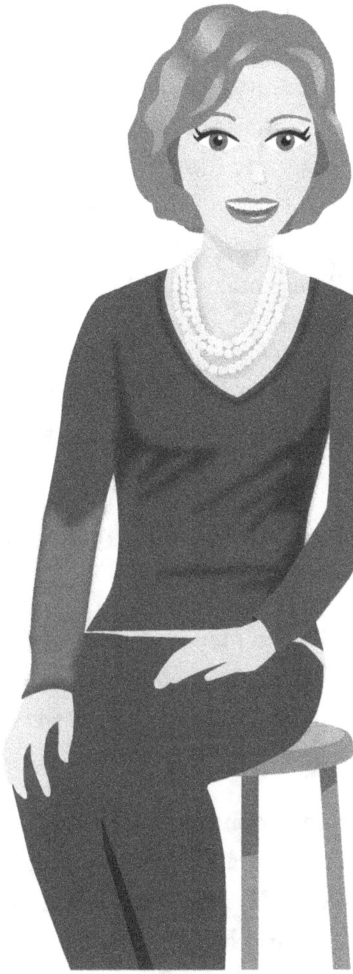

Do you worry about not finishing everything on time during an onsite monitoring visit? What will happen if you are disrupted by a crisis? Do you fret about whether you have covered all the regulatory and protocol requirements during your visit? If so, you are not alone.

Thinking about all the tasks that need to be done and all the documents that need to be reviewed can feel overwhelming. Experienced monitors learn to juggle many tasks and keep them all organized. Being clear about setting priorities—which tasks should be completed first, second, and third—will bring structure and order to this long list of tasks. The priorities at one visit may not be as important at the next visit. For example, you may check safety data at every visit but review regulatory documents at every other visit. In addition to the priority list, it is helpful to have a backup plan in case the priorities shift. Planning ahead will help make the best use of your time and the site's time during each monitoring visit.

As you focus on how to prioritize for monitoring visits, start with the basic activities that absolutely have to be done and build a list from there.

*Tasks and documents are the two main areas you need to prioritize during a site visit.*

**Tasks.** Identify all the tasks you plan to do while at the site. Some tasks are more important than others, some take more time, and some could be done if time allows. List the tasks for each site visit and prioritize them before arriving so you have a plan for the day.

**Documents.** With so many documents for every study, it is tempting to just start working when you walk in the door and trudge through as many tasks as you can in one day. However, it is much better to identify the most critical documents and confirm that those are checked during the monitoring visit.

## My Story about Prioritizing

I was monitoring at a location three-hour's drive from my office. I had sent a letter confirming the visit, called the day before to confirm the start time, and left my home at 6:00 a.m. When I arrived at 9:00 a.m., I was told that the study coordinator was not in the office. I got a cup of tea, reviewed my notes, pulled out my spreadsheets, and he was still not available. So, I asked the receptionist to page him. By 9:45 a.m. it was clear there was a problem and I was not going to be meeting with the coordinator that day. The receptionist tried to locate the PI, but he was not available either. Since I had driven a long distance to the site, I felt compelled to make productive use of my time. Fortunately, I had a backup plan.

I expected to review safety data, but I was not allowed access to the charts without the study coordinator. By moving to my backup plan, I was still able to review three areas that day: regulatory documents, investigational product, and the laboratory facilities. I connected with a nurse in the back office who provided access to the regulatory binder. I worked with the research pharmacist and reviewed investigational product accountability records. And finally, I met the laboratory director and discussed collection of laboratory specimens for this trial. By knowing how to re-prioritize when events took an unexpected turn, I was able to make good use of my time and justified my site visit. However, I still had the problem of the missing coordinator to solve.

I spoke with the PI the next day and learned that the coordinator, burdened with work, had not completed the CRFs. Being unprepared, he was reluctant to meet with me, so he left the building. The PI and I negotiated that I would coach the coordinator through the first few pages of the CRFs by telephone and reschedule a monitoring visit. The PI guaranteed me the coordinator would be available at my next visit.

*Here are suggestions on how to prioritize your tasks during a monitoring visit:*

**Put people before data.** The members of the site staff are members of your team. An essential part of good monitoring is building good teams. Interacting well with the people at the site is extremely important, so take the time to be friendly and cooperative with each of them. Connect with every key individual every time you visit the site. Schedule part of your day to interface with the people and to handle whatever issues arise. There are many courses and workshops on building effective teams and successfully interacting with people. I encourage you to add this competence to your skill set.

**Have a plan.** Create a strategic plan for each site visit. It may be similar each time, but clinical trials are very dynamic, so your strategy for each unique site will change as needed. The strategy will help you create mini goals for the day and allow you to be successful at meeting those goals. One approach I use is to set a target for the number of charts I will review and see if I can achieve that number.

**Focus on what you are being paid to do.** Focus on the activities in your job description. This is a very business-like approach and will help you eliminate time-wasting activities.

**Think about how much you are paid per minute.** Whether you work for a sponsor or a contract research organization (CRO), calculate how much you are being paid by the minute. With this monetary value in mind, ask yourself, "If I was paying myself this much per minute to do the work, would I be getting the most for my money?"

**Determine how much time each task will take.** As you create a priority list, estimate how much time each task takes. In this dynamic, ever-changing world of clinical investigation, the time required to perform a task will change based upon the project and the stage of the project. For example, it might take longer to review regulatory documents at the beginning of the study than at the end, but reviewing drug accountability may take longer later in the trial.

**Make priority lists and backup lists.** List all the tasks that need to be done at the site. (Don't forget to include the reviewing of charts, investigational products, facilities, and equipment. These, among other activities, need to be conducted in person to ensure their continued acceptability for the clinical research study.) From this all-inclusive list, consider the activities that are the highest priority. Estimate the amount of time required to do the highest priority tasks. Once the highest priority tasks are accomplished, move to other less pressing areas and spend time on those. A skilled monitor will always have a plan for prioritizing the work at the site and a plan for reprioritizing should unexpected events occur.

*Here are suggestions on how to prioritize the review of all documents during a monitoring visit:*

**Safety.** My firm rule is "always look at safety first." Patient safety is of utmost concern. Find ways to prioritize chart review for safety events first, especially if there has been a safety event since your last visit. Review all the forms and documents related to that safety event. Ask the coordinator questions to clarify the outstanding data points. Ensure that the site has processed the required forms according to the protocol, the site's standard operating procedures (SOPs), the IRB requirements, and the applicable regulations.

**Consent forms.** The second priority is usually the patients' rights and well-being, so ensure that the signed consent forms for any new patient are available and correct. Errors in consent forms are one of the most common findings during audits and inspections. The consent forms are often in the files but are incorrect in some way. Frequently, the wrong version was used, the patient did not sign or date the consent form correctly, or it cannot be determined that consent was obtained prior to any investigational procedures being performed. There are lots of details that must be reviewed in order to ensure proper consent was obtained. Take time to look carefully at each new consent form and accurately record your findings.

**Newly completed CRFs and corresponding medical chart.** For recently completed CRFs, make it a high priority to check the data against the subject's permanent medical records. Even if there is an EDC system, the accuracy of the data needs to be ensured. Be sure to identify any discrepancies. Checking CRF data against permanent medical record (PMR) data are one of the most time consuming tasks of monitoring. Remember, if you don't catch errors, the error may never be caught, because you may be the only one besides the coordinator who ever reviews the original data points. Errors that are undetected during monitoring can have serious repercussions if the FDA reviews data and finds errors such as the new drug application (NDA) or the premarket approval (PMA) being delayed. Monitors have a very serious responsibility to accurately verify all required data.

**Investigational product accountability records.** Investigational product is always critical to the study, so plan to fit it in your review. Check the shipping manifest, the packaging, the labels, the temperature logs, the product accountability log, and expiration dates. Given that all these tasks related to study drugs or investigational devices must be done in person, make certain to allocate time at the site to examine the integrity of the investigational product and document all discrepancies. Be sure to account for all used and unused product. Ensure that there is an unbreakable chain of custody from the sponsor's investigational product shipment depot all the way to the patient.

**Recent regulatory documents.** Review of regulatory documents often fall at the bottom of the priority list, primarily because they can usually be viewed remotely. Most sites send electronic or hard copies of these documents to the monitor. If there are recent regulatory documents or if a sponsor requires that certain regulatory documents are always reviewed, time needs to be allocated to this activity.

**Other documents.** Once the most important documents are reviewed, others can be checked as time allows. These could include other essential documents, laboratory reports, IRB correspondence, or any other study-specific paperwork.

## Key to Success to Prioritize

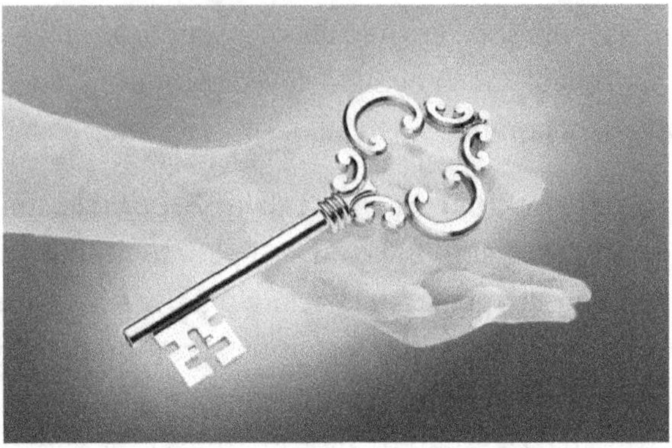

### Create a Priority Plan and a Backup Plan.

Instead of being overwhelmed by all the activities that need to be done during a monitoring visit, create a strategy for prioritizing tasks and documents. A priority plan will make the most of your time and exemplify your professionalism.

To be prepared for the unexpected, create a backup plan before you visit a site. You could base the backup plan on your experience with that particular site or the needs of the clinical team. It could include whom to contact if the coordinator is unavailable, what to review if the electricity goes off, or how to document information if you forget your power cord. Think through several potential scenarios when you make your backup plans. Since you can't think of everything, if an issue arises, you will be able to use your best judgment and still perform a solid monitoring visit. It ensures that you will make the best use of your time on site.

In this section I have provided ideas about how to create a priority plan and a backup plan before each monitoring visit to avoid becoming overwhelmed. While there is no specific way to manage your time or to set priorities, these ideas will help you use your time at the site as efficiently as possible. By creating priority plans and backup plans in advance, you will be more efficient, relaxed, and professional. Make the best use of your time, the site's time, and the company's money by setting priorities for each monitoring visit.

# Organize

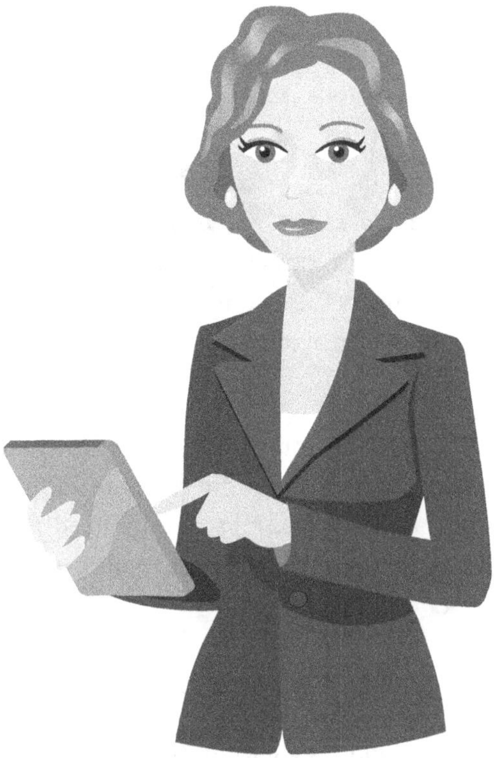

In the clinical research business, we see more data, receive and send more emails, and attend more meetings than ever before. With only a limited amount of time and energy each day, it is crucial to be organized.

The best way to be truly organized is to create a system and stick with it. In the beginning of my career, I asked more experienced monitors to share their tips on how to stay organized. By incorporating some of their ideas, I created a system that works well for me. As you experiment and gain experience, you will discover the methods that are best for you.

Some people are naturally well organized. Are you one of them?

Here's what I call the "closet test." Go to your closet and open the door. Are the slacks, shirts, and tops all arranged by category and color and neatly lined up on hangers? Are your shoes in labeled boxes? If so, then you are naturally well organized, and the job of monitoring will be easier for you.

If, however, when you open your closet you see chaos, then it is clear that you are less organized. The more disorganized you are, the more you need systems to help you find what you need and track what you have done. Ease, speed, and efficiency all result from a solid system to organize your work.

Once you determine an organizational system, use it consistently. There are lots of advantages to becoming proficient in your own system. You will be able to enter data more easily, know where to find information, and identify if something is out of place.

There are lots of tools to help you organize your work. You can find great ideas on the internet and in books. Make use of checklists, to-do lists, color-codes, charts, and other tools to manage your tasks and increase your productivity.

## My Story about Organizing

After about a year working as a CRA, I had the opportunity to move on to a more challenging project. The senior CRA in the new group had a reputation for being well organized, so I knew I would learn a lot from her. The second day on the job, I asked her about her filing system. This was at a time when there was one administrative assistant for every three senior staff members, so admittedly, she had a fair amount of help.

"Color is the key," she responded and then opened her file drawer. I was flabbergasted! She had organized her files with colored hanging file folders and matching colored file folders, all with typed labels. And there were no papers on her desk. I just stared. It was beautiful and so organized. I decided right then and there that this system would work for me and began to use it immediately.

There are two main areas for being organized: objects and time. Some of us are better at one than the other. Earlier you took the "closet test" to determine how well you organize objects. Now think about how well you use your time. Do you show up for meetings on time? Do you use a daily, weekly, and monthly calendar to stay on schedule? If you find that being on time is easy, congratulations! You manage your time effectively. If this is not your forte, time management tools will help you better track, plan, and organize your time.

To determine in what areas you need to build your organizational skills, analyze your current abilities to organize time and objects effectively and efficiently. Once you understand your shortcomings, use the following guidelines to help you improve your skills in the areas needed.

## Guidelines for Organizing Time

1. Use only one calendar
2. Never be on time
3. Think ahead
4. Block time

1. **Use only one calendar.** At one time, our family had three calendars: one in the kitchen, one in my office, and one in my husband's office. On one occasion, when I was out of town on a monitoring visit, I forgot about an event, and it became a family crisis. I learned a valuable lesson: we needed to consolidate all events on one electronic calendar. Since that time, by using only one calendar, I rarely miss a scheduled event.

2. **Never be on time.** Always be early! Yes, this little commitment helps me frequently. If I plan to be just on time, I don't have the few extra minutes that may be needed for an unexpected event. I plan to leave early so even if I run into traffic, I'll have ample time to handle additional setbacks (e.g. having to park blocks away from the site) and still arrive on time. If everything goes well and I am early, I use those few minutes to review my notes for the meeting or glance at the newspaper. I am not rushed, so I arrive at the appointment calm and prepared.

3. **Think ahead.** To stay organized, always look at the week ahead and the month ahead. First think about the big time-consuming tasks, then fit in the smaller activities around these big tasks. Plan the week on Sunday night or Monday morning. Look ahead to the next month and schedule the most important events first. Planning and thinking ahead is a big help to stay organized and efficient.

4. **Block time.** Setting aside blocks of time is an important time management skill. Determine the time needed for a task, such as writing a monitoring report or preparing for a meeting, and block that time on the calendar. Business trips can be extremely productive by using short blocks of time wisely. Before getting on a flight, be sure you have all the information on hand to complete a task. What a terrific feeling to have a project, the time to do it, and the completed document at the end of your trip.

## Guidelines for Objects

1. A place for everything and everything in its place
2. Like things stick together
3. Create a template once
4. Purge regularly
5. Make checklists
6. Create a color-coded system

1. **A place for everything and everything in its place.** Decide where you will keep an item and always place it there. For example, I always place my car keys in the same pouch in my purse. Even when I rent a car, those keys also go in the same pouch. I know my system works because I have never lost my car keys. If you use this practice to store any item, you will know where to find the item because it's always in the same place.

2. **Like things stick together.** This is one of my favorite organizational tips because it truly helps when I am sorting documents, using either electronic form or hardcopy. Put like things together and see how easy it is to find them. For example, if you have a supply cabinet at the office, notice how all the paperclips are easy to find and easy to put away because they are always in one bin.

3. **Create a template once.** Whenever I have a document or sections of a document that will be repeated, I create a template that can be used over and over again. For example, I have invested time and effort preparing several templates for follow-up letters. Then, when I complete a site visit, I simply choose the most appropriate follow-up letter template and tweak and edit it to personalize my new follow-up letter to the site personnel. It is very efficient.

4. **Purge regularly.** I reduce clutter by purging electronic files and paper documents regularly. For example, I delete unimportant emails on the same day received, sometimes at the moment one flies into my inbox. I also purge and shred duplicate or unnecessary paper documents so they don't clutter up my office.

5. **Make checklists.** Surgeons and pilots ensure that each step in a critical procedure is followed by using a checklist. This same rigor can be applied to monitoring. The saying "the devil is in the details" applies to the work of a CRA. Although paying attention to small details can seem tedious when there is so much to do, putting in that extra effort is critical. Otherwise, you may miss important information. Custom checklists will help ensure that you don't miss those details. For example, if there is a standard monitoring checklist supplied by the sponsor, use it. But, in addition, create your own spreadsheets to augment the monitoring checklist and to keep track of other details.

   You can use checklists to remind you about what to do ahead of the trip, during the trip, and after the trip. For example, it is helpful to have a checklist with a list of questions to ask the site personnel at the end of the monitoring visit. As you go through the regulatory binder, you might flag a question for the PI with a blue flag and then note the question on the questions checklist. During your meeting, you can show the PI the area in question (which is easily found with the blue flag) and then check off the answer on your questions checklist. If the answer is not known, it becomes an action item, and you can copy this action item from the checklist to the Action Item Table. This questions checklist is useful to document and resolve important issues.

6. **Create a color-coded system.** Color code your files so you can quickly spot the ones you want. Assign a color to each key area that you need to monitor and then create strategic files in the designated color. Here are some examples of the items that I color code:

- **Emails:** I use buttons to color code emails sent to and from each site so I can easily sort the emails by color and then identify them by topic.
- **Reminders:** Using the reminder application on my cell phone, I color code reminders according to the topic.
- **Sticky notes or flags:** During the monitoring trip, I use sticky notes or flags in the pre-designated colors. This is especially useful for flagging questions in the paper regulatory binders.
- **Paper folders:** I use colored file folders to identify key documents that cannot be stored electronically. This makes it easy to quickly find the correct folder on my desk or in my briefcase.
- **Index cards or reminder applications:** I use color-coded index cards to note information about the main personnel at each site. This was a clever system I learned when I took a sales training class. The sales people used this technique to remember important facts about each customer. I adapted this system to track key facts about the staff at each of my sites. Choose a color for each person, use corresponding colored index cards, and start collecting information about each person on the cards. I jot down things I learn by phone, email, or in person so I can remember more about that individual. For example, I may learn that the PI and I went to the same college or that the CRC has two boys who play soccer. I write these details on the colored index card and refer to them prior to each monitoring visit. It helps me connect with each person on an individual level. If you don't want to use colored index cards, electronic methods—such as applications on smart phones—are available to capture this information

## Key to Success to Organize

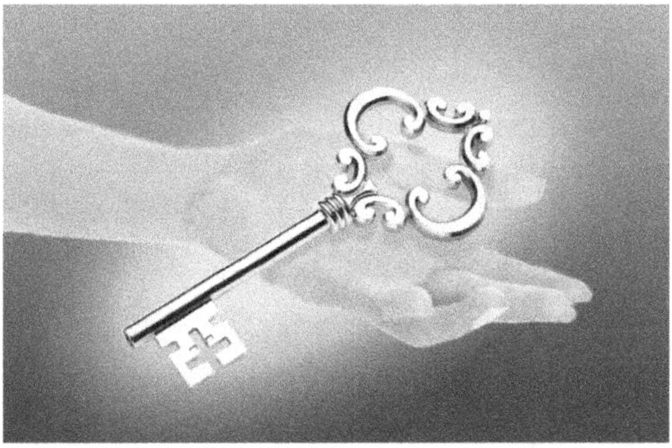

Color code all documents associated with each area.

I recommend selecting colors for various areas of monitoring and applying the selected colors to all emails, reminders, sticky notes, folders, and index cards for each monitoring site. The following colors are examples I use to differentiate the various areas of site monitoring:

PI = **blue** CRC = **yellow** Lab = **red**
Investigational Product = **green** Regulatory = **purple**

In this chapter, I presented various methods to organize time and objects, and I provided several examples of how you can apply these methods when monitoring clinical investigations. Using this information, I encourage you to analyze any gaps in your organizational skills and look for ways to improve your systems. These tips will help you to work smarter, not harder, and to accomplish your daily monitoring tasks more quickly and efficiently.

# Scrutinize

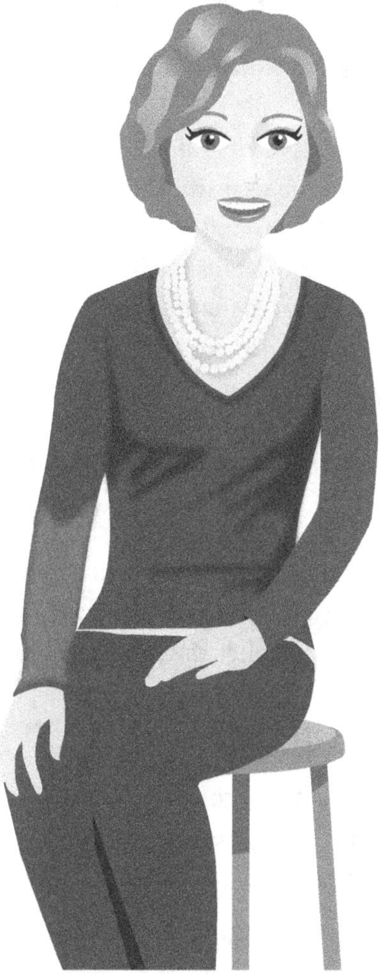

CRAs are overwhelmed with data, dates, addresses, signatures, time stamps, dosages, temperature logs, and more while performing on-site monitoring. To manage so much information well, attention to detail is essential.

Having a good eye for detail and scrutinizing all the numbers make it easier to keep track of details and to see when things are awry. Being meticulous can be a big advantage to a monitor.

Think of yourself as a detective—doing clinical investigation. Like any good detective, take the time to look at all the small details. The famous fictional detective Hercule Poirot never missed a clue. Whether it was a whiff of tobacco smoke or a minuscule thread on the floor, he was a master at details and solving the mystery. Be that kind of detective. Review the little details in charts, regulatory documents, product accountability forms, signatures, laboratory reports and all the other data you observe. Look for patterns, find consistency or inconsistency, see the logical flow of data, and identify accuracy of visit dates and dosing schedules as you investigate the clinical trial. With this approach, as you review the data for each subject in the study, you can identify potential errors.

Why is it so important to scrutinize data carefully? Data are the bottom line for clinical trials. Accurate data are used to prove safety and efficacy and to determine whether the product is marketable. The whole goal of performing clinical trials is to help future patients with safe and effective drugs and devices.

When we check the data thoroughly, we can identify protocol violations, inappropriate dosing regimens, incorrect screening procedures, and potential fraud.

I highly recommend that monitors read the chart first, then review the data entered on the CRFs. It is important to see the "story" for each subject in the context of the chart notes before looking at the CRFs. By doing this, the small inconsistencies pop out in a way they wouldn't have otherwise.

## My Story about Scrutinizing

One of my first bosses in my monitoring career was a very picky person. She was perfect. Her desk was always tidy and she did not have a hair out of place. She went out to a site with me and trained me how to monitor. I looked at charts, data, regulatory documents and investigational product. Near the end of the day, she reviewed my work. She scanned the checklists and then started to ask me some questions. "Why doesn't the dispensing date match the visit date on this subject, why doesn't the lab address on the Form FDA 1572 match the lab report form, and why did you check that this subject qualified when the chart indicates they had surgery last month?" Well, I thought I was paying attention to the details, looking at all the dates, data, numbers, and addresses, but clearly it was not at the level of detail required in this business. My lesson learned the hard way was to slow down, not assume I knew it all, pay even closer attention to detail, and constantly scrutinize so as not to miss these discrepancies.

| Examples of Problems and Results from Site Errors | |
|---|---|
| **Problem** | **Result** |
| Subjects enrolled in violation of the protocol | High numbers of protocol violations could result in poor quality data. The study may not meet its endpoints or the enrolled subjects might be placed at risk. |
| Subjects given the incorrect dose of study drug or incorrect use of medical device | Incorrect dosing of drugs or use of devices could result in adverse events or even death for study participants. |
| Site screening incorrect types of subjects | Inappropriate screening could result in the site enrolling unqualified subjects, which increases the time and cost of the study. |
| Perfect data | Data that are too good to be true is a potential sign of falsified data and possible fraud. Finding fraud at a site has an enormous ripple effect on the clinical trial, the site, and the sponsor. |

As you review the charts, make notes to help you remember key dates or facts and check off key points such as subject entry criteria, dates of visits, and dispensing dates. However, remember that just because you jot down notes on your personal spreadsheet these notes are not copied into the monitoring report or follow-up letter.

Be very exacting about all the numbers you review. Try to ensure that good documentation practices are followed, such as:

1. A consistent date format is used
2. The appropriate individuals have access to the electronic systems
3. All signatures have names typed or printed beneath them
4. The appropriate individuals have signed the documents
5. Every signature is dated or date stamped electronically by the person who signed the document
6. Every page has a page number
7. Every page is labeled to identify the purpose of the document and the study, whether it is electronic or paper
8. Every blank field is filled in

One document that is frequently problematic is the Delegation of Authority (DoA) Log form. This form is not required by regulation; however, many sponsors have adopted its use to identify which individuals at the site were involved in the study and the dates of their involvement. Each sponsor or CRO may have a slightly different form, but every field should be completed and it should be kept up to date at all times. Review this form and confirm good documentation practices are followed.

Check data early in the study when the first few subjects are enrolled so you can see trends and catch common errors so they won't be repeated throughout the clinical trial. If you find problems in the beginning, address them quickly—either before you leave the site or within a few days of the monitoring visit. By identifying problems as soon as possible, you will help the site to perform a cleaner and more error-free study. Scrutinize information on the CRFs and in the subject's permanent medical record to identify errors before small problems become larger ones.

Regardless of whether you are well organized by nature or need a lot of systems in place, everyone benefits from methods of keeping all the data and facts organized and available.

During a recent monitoring visit I used a spreadsheet to record the subject numbers, enrollment dates, and visit dates before performing investigational product accountability. For the second subject I reviewed, a drug dispensing date seemed odd. When I saw it, I immediately checked my notes and noticed that the pharmacist had transposed the date. I discussed it with the pharmacist and the problem was resolved that day. This error might have been caught during data cleanup but it was quite helpful for the site and the project to resolve the problem sooner rather than later.

## Key to Success to Scrutinize

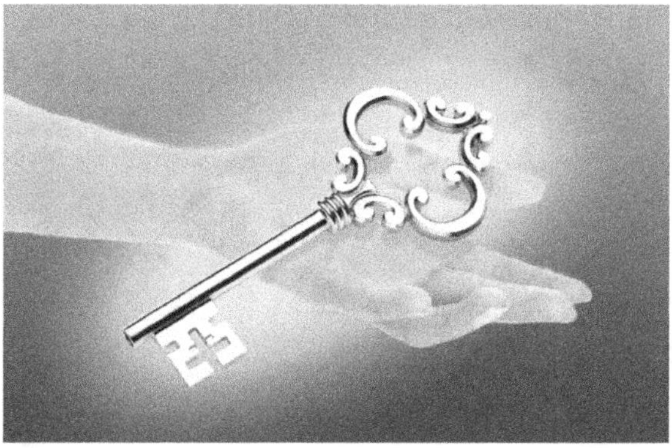

### Create a Zip List spreadsheet.

This contains all the key variables and documents that should be reviewed at each monitoring visit. As you go through the charts and files, check off each item. Scrutinize all the data. This is your own personal documentation of what was reviewed and this list will help you identify the gaps that need to be filled in before you leave the site. Of course, you will not be writing down every data point. A list of key parameters—such as visit dates, subject numbers, and dosing requirements—will help you immensely.

We have discussed how all the data can be overwhelming in a clinical trial and why it is imperative for monitors to pay close attention to the details. Be meticulous when reviewing every date, address, dosage, and chart note.

Try your powers of observation on the next airplane flight. How many seats are unoccupied? How many baseball caps, maxi dresses, and babies do you notice? Pay attention to what you see daily and this will help you develop a keener eye and a heightened sense of attention to detail in everyday activities as well as in monitoring.

Create a system as you review key data points and check them off as you go. Scrutinize the information as if you were a detective and this will result in higher quality data and a cleaner data set for all the trials you monitor.

# Follow Up

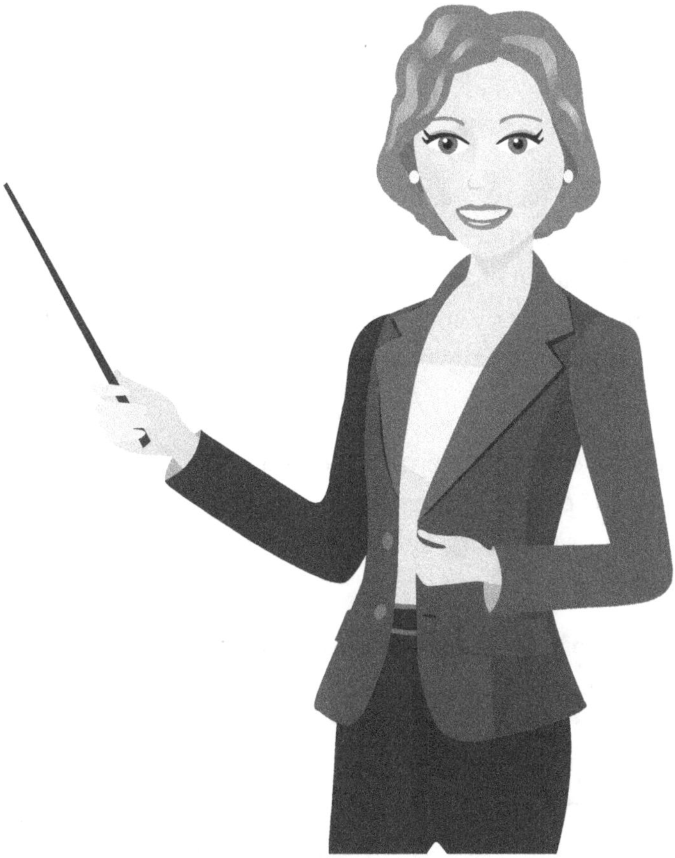

There is a saying in clinical research: "If it isn't documented, it didn't happen," and it is usually the monitor's responsibility to obtain documents to prove it happened!

In order to do this, you need to ask PIs, coordinators, colleagues, IRBs, auditors, managers, and many others to document all the actions they have taken related to the clinical trial.

This could be documenting a decision that was made or signing a form, but all of these actions must be either written down on paper or captured electronically.

In this section I will emphasize the importance of following up on requests, and I will describe techniques to ensure the follow-up action is documented. Documentation is critical, but there is more. The documents must be clearly and accurately recorded according to good documentation practices, signed off by the appropriate individual, and filed in the right location.

To totally finish monitoring at a site, you need to confirm that the follow-up work is complete on every outstanding action item related to that visit. This is one of the hardest things to do, but also one of the most important.

As the monitor, you should set a good example by following up on the site's requests as soon as possible after a monitoring visit. If the coordinator needs a question answered, more investigational product sent, or more supplies shipped, do your best to finish the request quickly. My personal goal is to complete all requests within 24 hours of the visit. I try to get the task done or at least started the very next day. It sets such a good example for the team. It's a wonderful modus operandi, and it sets the standard that if you do it for them, they will do it for you.

Once you complete the task, notify the site. And if this task is not something that you can perform personally, such as sending more investigational product, let the site know as soon as you have made the request. Of course, always follow up to see that each request was properly handled, such as ensuring the next shipment of investigational product was sent promptly and arrived in good condition.

## My Story about Following Up

I was training a monitor who had been an in-house CRA for about three years, but she had little experience in the field. We were closing a database and needed to ensure that all the queries were completed and the corresponding data were recorded in the permanent medical record. The former monitor had quit suddenly, leaving us with several outstanding safety parameters to find, and so we took this opportunity to go to the site and collect this data. After looking through charts, checking data, and meeting with the coordinator, we still had two subjects with missing safety data. We had to leave for the day, but the coordinator assured us that he would send the data within the next 24 hours.

On the plane home, we discussed the trip, and I asked the monitor what she would do to follow up. "Well, he said he would send the data from those two subjects, so I am sure he will," was the reply. I told her that she was in charge of getting the data, and I recommended she send the coordinator an Action Item Plan to clearly outline the steps, the documents, and the timeline that we had agreed upon.

Two days later I stopped by the CRA's desk to see the results. The database closure was imminent. Everyone was working frantically, but we did not have the safety data yet. "We need to talk about how to actually get that data, because it is vital to the safety information," I stated. I sat down with the CRA, and we discussed all the ways she could try to obtain that information. She said she would call and email the coordinator, but if that didn't work, she didn't know what else to do. Since we were in a time crunch and nothing was forthcoming from the site I told her that going "up the ladder" usually worked. Eventually, this was what she decided to do. With pressure from the sponsor's medical monitor applied to the PI, we finally received the pertinent data, and the queries were closed. The CRA told me that she learned the value of setting up an Action Item Table—sooner, not later—so that everyone was clear about the follow-up steps required.

In order to keep track of the requests from each site, create an electronic Action Item Table. Some strategies to create successful tables are as follows:

1. Describe the action accurately and specifically so that anyone who reads the table will know what is needed.
2. List the estimated and actual completion dates. Everyone responds more quickly to a deadline.
3. Include information about how the issue was resolved. It may prove useful if similar situations arise in the future.

- **Specify your actions.** For example, here is a vague action: Update Form 1572. And here is a specific action: Obtain new address of Hamilton Clinical Laboratory, update Form 1572 with this address in section 4, have Dr. J.P. sign form, and send electronically to P. Kasper.
- **Action item.** For each new request, create a new action item on a separate line in the Action Item Table. State what needs to be accomplished in a clear, concise, complete sentence.
- **Dates.** A key to clear communication is to agree on the expected completion date for each action item. The completion date should be shortly after the monitoring visit. Negotiate the completion date for all action items to be within a few days of your visit, if possible. The advantage is that you may be able to note all the action items as completed in the follow-up letter—which finishes your visit and makes you and the coordinator look good.
- **Documenting the completion of actions.** Copy the Action Item Table from the monitoring report and insert it in the follow-up letter to the site. If all actions are completed, there is no additional work to be done. If actions need to be completed after the follow-up letter is sent, either mention them in an email or in the letter confirming the next monitoring visit. In this way, the completed items are documented in monitoring visit reports and in the communication to the site.

If there is an action item that is particularly problematic, it may be dealt with separately. When it is finally resolved, you need to document the resolution in a letter, a note-to-file, an email, or other appropriate manner.

And finally, if there is a task that just can't seem to be resolved, you are apparently not approaching the problem correctly. Either the timing is not realistic, the individual assigned to complete the task is the wrong person, or there is some other reason for not getting the issue resolved. In this case, "go up the ladder" and work with the PI at the site, your director, the medical monitor, or someone else at a higher level who has the power to actually make it happen. These are unique cases, and experience will show you how to get past the roadblock.

## Key to Success to Follow Up

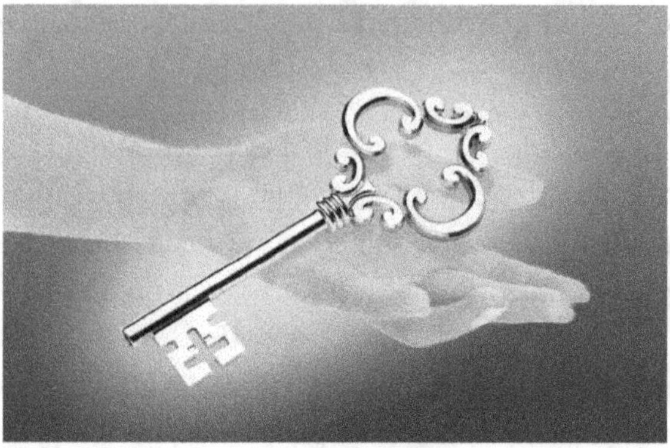

### Create an Action Item Table after every site monitoring visit.

A weakness of many monitors is not following up consistently and effectively on **all** the issues identified during a site visit. The tools described in this section will help you understand how to capture the issue clearly, set a date for completion, and make sure the proper documentation is completed for each action item. By putting this kind of plan in place, you will communicate unambiguously what is needed from the site and have a clear audit trail for all issues that arose and were resolved during the entire clinical study.

## Example Agenda*

### Dr. J.P. San Diego, CA, Study XYZ Site 621
### Monitoring Visit 9/10-9/11/2012

| Action | Person Responsible | Date Expected | Date Completed | How Resolved |
|---|---|---|---|---|
| Sign protocol amendment #2 cover page & send to sponsor | Dr. J.P. Principal Investigator | 9/18/12 | 9/12/12 | Stephen H. brought page to weekly CRC team meeting, obtained signature, & sent to sponsor |
| Return all used vials to sponsor for completed patients | Stephanie M., Pharmacist | 9/18/12 | TBD | TBD |
| Create list of additional blood tubes needed | Stephen H., CRC | 9/11/12 | 9/11/12 | Stephen H. created list & emailed to P. Kasper during site visit |

*All names in this example are fictional.

# Consequences of Improper Monitoring: Pfizer Warning Letter

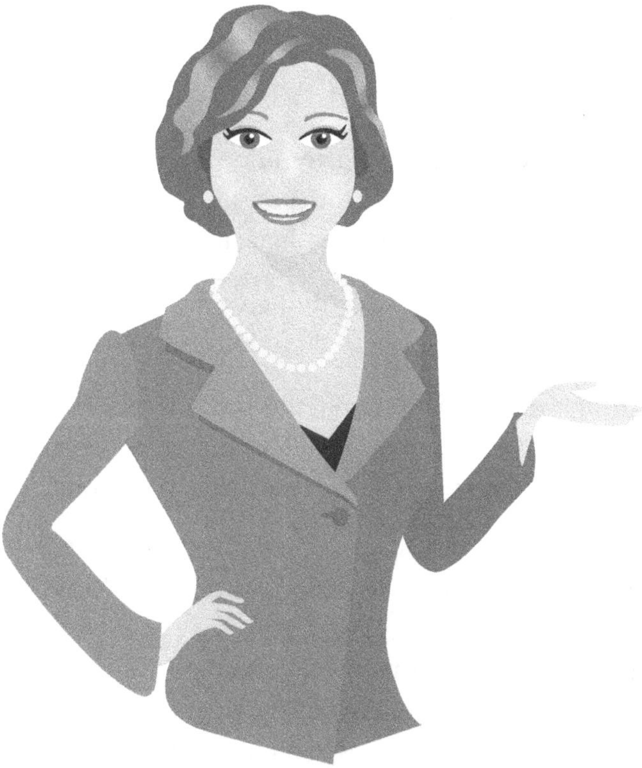

It is unfortunate when problems arise in the development of a new drug or device. Often, these problems are not known publically because the company solves them internally.

However, all warning letters are published on the FDA's website (www.fda.gov), and when a corporation receives a warning letter, it is available to everyone.

In April 2010, Pfizer Corporation received a warning letter from the FDA. The company was cited for failure to:

- ensure proper monitoring of the clinical investigation. [21 CFR 312.50]
- ensure that the investigations were conducted in accordance with the general investigational plan and protocols contained in the IND. [21 CFR 312.50]
- keep the participating investigator informed of new observations discovered by or reported to the sponsor on the drug, particularly with respect to adverse effects and safe use. [21 CFR 312.55(b)]

In this chapter, I will focus only on the first citation: "failure to ensure proper monitoring of the clinical investigation."

By using the information from this warning letter that is publicly available on http://www.fda.gov/ICECI/EnforcementActions/WarningLetters/ucm208976.htm, we are able to see some important consequences of improper monitoring.

This was a repeat violation of findings communicated to Pfizer in April 2005 following an FDA inspection. The patient population was pediatric patients being treated with the antipsychotic drug Geodon for bipolar disorder and schizophrenia. The FDA letter states: "As a result of inadequate monitoring, widespread overdosing of study subjects at multiple study sites was neither detected nor corrected in a timely manner. Study monitors failed to ensure that the investigation was conducted in accordance with the investigational plan. Overdosing at one site was neither recognized nor reported by study monitors in a timely manner."

The monitoring occurred on the following dates:

- March 13 & 15
- April 25
- May 15-16
- June 6-7
- July 5-6

This frequency of monitoring appears to be sufficient to determine that the site was following the protocol and complying with GCP; however, dosing errors occurred and overdosing extended over several days for seven pediatric subjects—in one case for as long as 22 days.

The reason for the failure to identify these dosing errors is unknown. It could be postulated that the monitors were busy, lacked proper training, did not utilize proper monitoring tools, or were not well supervised. Whatever the case, the reason doesn't matter to us; the consequences do. In this example, we can identify and examine the consequences in each area and learn from them.

Improper monitoring affects the subjects, the PI, the sponsor, and the data in this trial.

The subjects were affected because they could experience serious adverse events as a result of overdosing. Their rights were violated because they did not receive the care that they had agreed to in the informed consent. Pediatric patients probably signed an assent form, and their parent or guardian signed the consent form. In that case, the parents were affected as well as the patients. All of this could have been avoided with proper monitoring.

The PI was affected because he or she did not adhere to the agreement with the sponsor and with the FDA in conducting the protocol according to GCP. The PI put the patients at risk unnecessarily. Physicians generally adhere to high standards in the treatment of patients and would not want to see any of their patients put at risk. The site personnel will probably also need to correct these errors and that will take time and resources, and they may not be compensated for this extra effort. The PI and the site may experience future audits by FDA. They may need to implement procedures to ensure this does not happen in the future. All these tasks could have been eliminated with proper monitoring from the sponsor and training for the site.

Pfizer, the sponsor, was affected; the company received a warning letter about the issue and had to rectify this situation. There could be even further reaching consequences to Pfizer, such as more site inspections, more sponsor inspections, and more interaction with FDA about this issue. This will all take time, money, and resources that would not have been needed if the monitoring had identified these errors earlier.

The data may be affected. Data from these overdosed patients could be in question. There will need to be decisions made about whether or not to include some of these data and/or how to explain the data in the clinical study report. This will take extra time and effort by the data management group, the biostatistics department, the medical monitors, and others.

The subjects, the PI, the sponsor, and the data are all affected by inadequate monitoring. As you can see, monitoring, whether good or bad, has a ripple effect. By analyzing the specific issues that were omitted, by assuming some of the causes of the problems, and by realizing the consequences of these actions, it is easier to see how good tools and techniques are crucial in monitoring.

# Conclusion

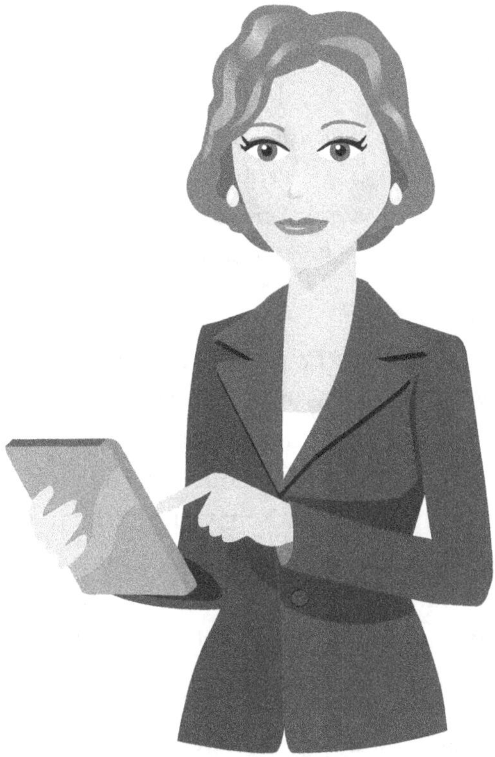

I hope that by reading this book you have found suggestions, tools, hints, tips, and ideas to improve your skills as a monitor of clinical trials.

*Here is a summary of the topics covered in this book:*

- **Before going to the site.** If you anticipate and prepare well before going to the site, you will increase your professionalism, enhance your credibility and increase your efficiency.
- **At the site.** Once at the site, use the tools provided in this book to prioritize activities and make the best use of your valuable time. Organize data as they are examined. Data review is of utmost importance in clinical trials so, scrutinize the data carefully. Remember, you may be the only one to find discrepancies. You want to be an exceptionally effective monitor in the time allotted for each visit.
- **After the site visit.** Follow up on the outstanding action items identified during the visit and you will excel in your job as a monitor. By creating and completing the action item list, you will be a strong contributor to the team, and your studies will run more smoothly. My goal in writing this book is to help you succeed in your career by providing you with proven ideas based on my personal experiences as a monitor. I encourage you to try these techniques. Your job will be easier and you will become more professional and more efficient in all of your monitoring activities.

To test your understanding of the importance of efficient, effective monitoring, complete the following three quiz questions.

## Skills Assessment

Test your understanding of some situations that you may see in the field. For each of the questions below, choose the best answers. Please note there may be more than one correct answer.

### Question #1

What are ways to document that the consent was obtained prior to any clinical trial procedure being done?

a. The CRC enters the time of consent in the eCRFs.

b. The CRC shows the monitor the SOP stating that consent is required prior to any clinical trial procedures.

c. The CRC documents time of consent in PMR.

d. The patient documents time of consent next to their signature on the consent.

**Answer:** The best answers are a, c, and d. All of these techniques would be actual proof of when the patient read and accepted the consent for that specific trial. There is no regulation that states the time the consent was signed needs to be documented; however, it is an excellent way to ensure that there is clear documentation that the consent was, in fact, obtained before any clinical trial procedures were initiated. Answer "b" is not correct because just having an SOP does not mean the procedure was done correctly and does not actually document the necessary data.

### Question #2

Why is identification of each protocol violation so important?

a. Entering non-eligible patients may expose them to unreasonable risks.

b. The sponsor may pay for worthless data from these patients.

c. The Investigator will be fined by the FDA for each protocol violation.

d. The Investigator may be cited by regulatory authorities for failure to follow the protocol.

**Answer:** The correct answers are a, b, and d. We need to be diligent about identifying protocol violations throughout the time a clinical trial is conducted because (a) we do not want to expose patients to unreasonable risk, (b) the data may be worthless, and (c) it is against regulation. At this point in time, the FDA do not fine sites for protocol violations.

### Question #3

Why should the monitor write a clear, succinct monitoring report?

a. It is how the sponsor knows what is happening at the site.

b. It helps the monitor track what was done previously.

c. It shows oversight and collaboration between the sponsor and the site.

d. It is required by FDA regulation 21 CFR 312.56(a).

**Answer:** The correct answers are a, b, and c. Clear, succinct reports do keep the sponsor informed of the activities at the site, help the monitor track previous actions and documents oversight of the site by the sponsor. However, a monitoring report is not required by this regulation. There is little information in the FDA regulations to tell us exactly how to report findings after a monitoring visit. Instead, we rely on the ICH E6 Guideline as well as industry standards and guidelines that have evolved over the years.

# Selected Resources for Clinical Research Monitors

## Associations

Association of Clinical Research Professionals (ACRP)
www.acrpnet.org

Drug Information Association (DIA)
www.diahome.org

Society of Clinical Research Associates (SoCRA)
www.socra.org

## Relevant Regulations & Guidance for Drug & Device Studies

- Food and Drug Administration (FDA) www.fda.gov
- Code of Federal Regulations (CFR) Title 21: Food & Drugs
- Part 11: Electronic Records: Electronic Signatures
- Part 50: Protection of Human Subjects
- Part 54: Financial Disclosure by Clinical Investigators
- Part 56: Institutional Review Boards
- Part 312: Investigational New Drug Application
- Part 314: Applications for FDA Approval to Market a New Drug
- Part 812: Investigational Device Exemptions
- Part 814: Premarket Approval for Medical Devices International Conference on Harmonisation (ICH) www.ich.org

- E2A: Clinical Safety Data Management: Definitions and Standards for Expedited Reporting
- E3: Structure and Content of Clinical Study Reports
- E6: Good Clinical Practice: Consolidated Guideline
- E8: General Considerations for Clinical Trials
- E9: Statistical Considerations in the Design of Clinical Trials International Standards Organization (ISO) www.iso.org
- ISO 14155: Clinical investigation of medical devices for human subjects — Good Clinical Practice

# About the Author

## Patricia O. Kasper, MS, CCRA

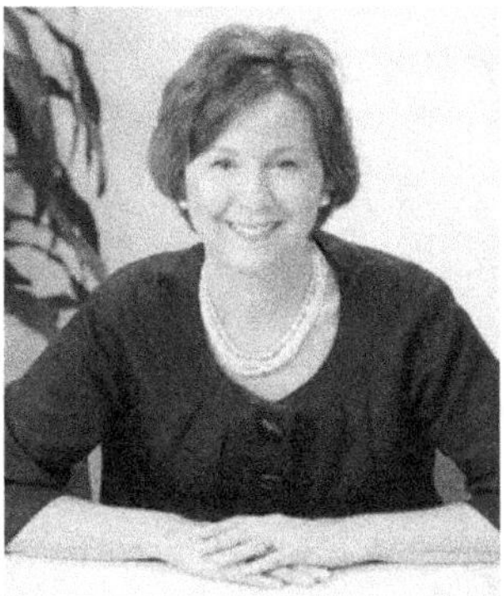

Patty Kasper is a recognized expert in clinical research training and operations with more than 20 years of industry experience. Since founding P. Kasper & Associates in 1995, Patty and her team of experienced professionals have provided expert consulting services to over 30 drug and device companies. Patty has led this team in providing well-designed training programs to the biopharmaceutical and medical device industries. More than 1300 professionals have benefitted from the hallmark hands-on interactive learning modules that bring an exciting real-world element to these classes. She has been on the faculty of UC Santa Cruz Extension as part of their prestigious Clinical Trials Design and Management Certificate Program.

Patty has direct experience with Phase 1-4 clinical research trials in numerous indications and has directed studies in the US, Canada and Europe. She has been involved with medical device trials and registry studies during her career.

Patty earned her Masters of Science degree from Washington State University. She is a medical technologist and a certified clinical research associate through the Association of Clinical Research Professionals.

www.ingramcontent.com/pod-product-compliance
Lightning Source LLC
LaVergne TN
LVHW022313200926
848481LV00004B/1314

* 9 7 8 0 9 8 6 2 1 9 1 1 5 *